Essential Oils For Family Health

Simple Aromatherapy Recipes For
Common Ailments

CORAL MILLER

ISBN-13:978-1512050233

ISBN-10:1512050237

TABLE OF CONTENT

Read Other Books By Coral Miller

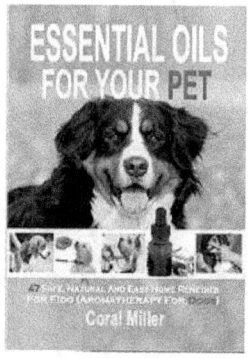

Essential Oils For Your Pet: 47 Safe, Natural And Easy Home Remedies For Fido (Aromatherapy for Dogs)

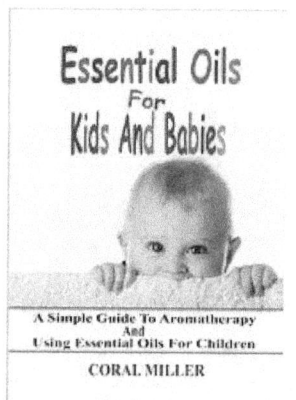

Essential Oils For Kids And Babies: A Simple Guide To Aromatherapy And Using Essential Oils For Children

INTRODUCTION

Essential oils are the potent and aromatic liquids extracted from the leaves, seeds, fruits, barks, flowers, roots or seeds of plants, herbs and shrubs. Essential oils are generally created through distillation, a process which separates the oil and water- based plant compounds by steaming.

Essential oils are highly concentrated oils with a strong aroma. Being highly concentrated, just one drop is sufficient to create powerful health benefits. What this means is that we are literally separating the most powerful healing compounds of a particular plant into one single oil. For example, to get a pound of lavender essential oil will require 150 pounds of lavender flowers! Do you see how highly concentrated essential oils are? So essentially (no pun meant), you will be getting 150 times the healing properties from lavender essential oils than you would get from using straight lavender.

The reason why these natural oils are in plants in the first place is to protect them (the plant) from insects and a harsh environment. So when you take essential oils, you will be harnessing the plant's healing and protective powers. Of a truth, essential oils are the most potent form of plant based medicine. So effective is their power to heal

1

and cure diseases that a lot of people can now successfully avoid taking a plethora of medications or undergoing various surgeries simply by taking essential oils correctly.

Why Essential Oils Are So Powerful

Essential oils are made of tiny molecules that can penetrate your cells. Some compounds in certain essential oils can even cross the blood-brain barrier. Fatty oils from vegetables or nuts come from large molecules so they cannot penetrate your cells. As a result, they are not therapeutic in any way. Unlike essential oils, vegetable oils are not small enough to get into your system so they can only stay on your skin and may end up even clogging your pores.

Essential oils are transdermal. When placed anywhere on the body, they pass through the skin and straight into the circulatory system and cells. They are so powerful that they are often diluted with a carrier oil such as coconut or olive oil before they can be used. Since they can travel through the body and the air (via diffusion) at an incredibly rate, they have great health benefits.

Think about this: if you had peppermint leaves in your kitchen, you probably wouldn't be able to smell them from 12 feet away, could you? But if you are diffusing peppermint or cinnamon essential oils you will be able to smell them throughout your home!

The reason for this is the volatile compounds that are in essential oils moves through your olfactory system (your sense of smell) to your cells and into your blood stream within seconds. So if your child is ill, you can diffuse clove and frankincense essential oils in the air to aid quick recovery and to keep your entire family healthy.

Once these oil compounds are in your system, they can protect and heal your body in a variety of ways. This is what is known as aromatherapy: natural healing from essential oils. At this juncture, it will be safe to mention that medicinal tinctures and dried herbs can also heal. Ground ginger root and cinnamon have lots of health benefits as well. Eating healthy foods like fresh herbs and vegetables can also support healing. Nevertheless, in terms of compounds with the strongest concentrated healing properties, essential oils surpass them all.

Quality Of Essential Oils

Not all essential oils are created the same. In fact, most of them are potentially toxic and worthless to your health. There are four grades of essential oils:

1. Synthetic and Altered Oils are the lowest grade of oil. They are created in laboratory.

2. Natural and "Pure" Oils. They are the most commonly sold type of oils. They are usually over-processed so they lose their healing compounds.

3. Wellness Grade Essential Oils; these are steam distilled with healing compounds. The only setback is that they may have been sprayed with pesticides.

4. Certified Therapeutic Grade Essential Oils; these are the highest grade of essential oils with maximum healing properties.

Only the highest quality essential oils can promote healing. To create true quality essential oils, the quality of plants and the quality of processing are important. High quality plants must be planted in nutrient dense organic soil and must be harvested when their healing compounds are most available.

The next step should is to extract the oils using steam distillation or cold pressed and not chemicals. Finally, bottle the oils in dark glass containers to protect from sunlight and oxidation. Ensure you buy therapeutic grade and organic oils at all times when purchasing essential oils.

How To Use Essential Oils

There are 3 main ways essential oils can be used: topical, inhalation and internal.

Topical Use

This involves applying essential oils on the skin, either directly or directly. A few oils can be applied directly on the skin e.g. lavender but most oils must be mixed with a carrier oil before usage. Some of the best carrier oils include jojoba oil, coconut oil, olive oil, almond oil and pomegranate seed oil.

Key points of application on the body are:

- Behind ears

- Abdomen

- Neck

- Temples

- Soles and tops of feet

- Along spine

- Upper back

Other topical ways to use oils include:

<u>Baths</u>: essential oils can be used as aromatherapy baths.. This could help improve circulation, relax the body, relieve sore muscles, open airways, improve sleep and soothe the skin. It is best to mix the oils with bath salts, milk or sesame oil for quick dispersion. Failure to do this will cause the oils to float on water and even stick to your skin directly. Use soothing oils like lavender and eucalyptus. Additionally, the bath could either be a full body bath or foot bath.

<u>Compresses</u>: compresses work well for infections, bruises, aches and pains. Simply add your preferred essential oil to bowl of either hot or cold water. (It could be diluted with carrier, depending on the treatment). Dip a clean cloth in the water, wring it out and place on the affected area. Peppermint works real well for muscle aches and lavender is just great for infections.

<u>Salves</u>: to make salves, mix coconut oil, vitamin E oil, beeswax and essential oils. Store in a metal or glass container and rub as needed. Salves are very effective for cuts, scrapes, bruises or sore muscle.

<u>Massage</u>: Aromatherapy massage is another effective topical application. Make sure that you always dilute with suitable carrier oil.

Inhalation

Diffusion is another excellent way to use essential oil. You can either use diffusers or inhale the oil directly in hot water. Inhalations are highly effective for headaches, respiratory and sinus problems. Only ensure that you inhale for 2- 3 minutes at a stretch. Inhaling essential oils for too long can cause nausea, dizziness and headaches.

Internal Use

Internal use of essential oils can only be effective if pure therapeutic grade oils are used. Dosage and dilution is also dependent on the individual's age, size and health. However, it is best to consult your physician or nutritionist before ingesting any essential oil.

Ways by which essential oils can be taken internally include:

• Putting a few drops in an empty capsule and swallowing with water

• Putting 1-3 drops of oil to 1 teaspoon of coconut oil then consume.

• Adding 1-3 drops of oil to a glass of coconut milk, water or almond milk.

• Adding 1-3 drops of oil to 1 teaspoon of raw honey.

Top Essential Oils For Healing

Stock these six essential oils in your medicine cabinet and keep your family healthy all year long.

Tea Tree

Also called Melaleuca, tea tree is a powerful antifungal, antibacterial and antiseptic oil. It can be used topically to treat all sorts of skin problems. You only need a few drops diluted with a carrier oil and your cuts, scrapes, acne blemishes, insect bites, ringworm, warts, fungal infections, athletic foot and even dandruff will be eliminated. It can also help to boost the immune system. In some cases, it can even be used undiluted. It is found in a lot of skin care products.

<u>Uses</u>

• Mix 5 drops with 1 tablespoon of raw honey and use mixture as acne free -face wash.

• Apply to ringworm, Candida, athlete's foot or other fungal infections.

• Put directly on mosquito, spider or bug bites to detox poison.

• Add 5 drops to your favorite shampoo to reduce dandruff and to improve scalp health.

• Kick a cold or flu by gargling tea tree oil and water.

• Mix 2 teaspoon of melaleuca and water in a spray bottle for an all- purpose cleaner.

• Diffuse in the air to purify it of mold and allergens.

Lavender

One of the most versatile oils, lavender has antiviral and antibacterial properties and it is effective on cuts, bruises and general skin care. It doesn't always require a carrier oil and can be applied directly to the affected area. It is relaxing and uplifting, helping to balance hormones in women and generally reducing the stress hormones in the body.

Uses

• To relax the body and improve sleep, rub on neck in the evenings.

• To restore the body after a long day, add a few drops to your bath along with some Epsom salts.

• Put on your kids' cuts, bruises, scrapes, burns, rashes, and wounds.

• Diffuse in the air improve mood and relax.

• Use topically on neck to lower cholesterol& blood pressure or take as supplement.

Peppermint:

Peppermint is cooling; it stimulates the mind and increases mental alertness. For an instant cooling effect, simply dilute with a carrier and rub on your chest, back and neck. Peppermint oil wards off nausea, morning or motion sickness.

It reduces headaches and migraines to a large extent when applied to the temple. It has antimicrobial properties as well so also helps to freshen bad breath and treat digestive issues such as flatulence, indigestion and slow digestion.

<u>Uses</u>

• Mix with coconut oil or carrier oil of choice and rub topically on sore muscles.

• Diffuse it in air to improve energy and focus.

• To improve breathing and fight infections, rub on bottom of feet& chest

• Mix with baking soda and coconut oil for homemade toothpaste.

• Freshen breath, put 1 drop in clean water.

• To improve digestion & reduce nausea, take 1 drop in water.

Lemon

Lemon oil is effective in its ability to detox every part of the body. With its uplifting properties, it is also good for improved focus, concentration and to rejuvenate energy. It helps treat wounds and infections and acts as a powerful bug repellent.

<u>Uses</u>

• To freshen breath, put 1-2 drops in water.

• To promote cleansing & metabolism, take 1 drop as supplement three times daily.

• To uplift mood, diffuse to clean air and enjoy a nice citrus scent.

• Improve home smell by diffusing in the air.

• Rub on hands in instead of hand sanitizer for its antimicrobial benefits.

• Mix with baking soda as all- natural teeth whitener.

• Mix with olive oil and use as natural cleaning product.

Frankincense

A very powerful essential oil, frankincense was valued above gold in ancient times due its ability to treat all sorts of illnesses. Recent research has shown that it is even more effective than chemotherapy in shrinking tumors and killing cancer cells. It helps to reduce inflammation and improve immune function. It also fights infections, heals acne, sunspot and skin scarring.

<u>Uses</u>

• To improve immunity, rub topically on neck, chest, behind ears and to bottoms of feet.

• Apply to minor cuts for healing and pain relief.

• To reduce scars, age spots and stretch marks, dilute oil and apply once or twice a day.

• Use after a trauma to calm yourself.

• Rub topically on areas of joint pain

• To relieve stress and headaches, apply to temples with lavender.

• Add to baths for extra relaxation.

• Diffuse in air to reduce seasonal allergies

Eucalyptus

This is a powerful antiviral, antibacterial and antispasmodic oil that works on coughs, colds and allergies that affect breathing. To clear your nasal passages and lungs, just add a few drops to a vaporizer or to bowl of steaming water and inhale. It stimulates the immune system and loosens congested chest. Prevent a full cold also by using regularly during cold season.

COLDS & COUGHS

Cough Mixture

2 drops Eucalyptus oil

2 drops Lemon oil

3 tablespoons honey

<u>What To Do</u>

1. Mix the oil and honey together.

2. Use 1 teaspoon of this mixture in half a glass of warm water.

3. Sip slowly.

Vapor Rub

For chest congestion

5 drops peppermint oil

12 drops eucalyptus oil

1 ounce olive oil

5 drops thyme oil

<u>What To Do</u>

1. Add all ingredients to a glass bottle, shaking to mix well.

2. Massage gently into throat and chest.

3. Use daily and always before bed time.

Power Chest Rub

For Coughs & Chest Congestion

<u>Ingredients</u>

2 tbsp virgin coconut oil or Shea butter

7 drops Peppermint essential oil

1/3 cup jojoba or olive oil

2 drops Cedarwood essential oil

15 drops Eucalyptus essential oil

1 drop Thyme essential oil

<u>What To Do</u>

1. Pour 1 inch water (2.5cm) in a medium-sized pot bottom and heat on low until it simmers.

2. Place the coconut oil or Shea butter in Pyrex or measuring cup. Place the Pyrex in the water and warm gently on low heat until the butter melts.

3. Remove from the heat, add the olive or jojoba oil and stir.

4. Pour the oil mixture into a PET or dark glass jar. Add the essential oils.

5. Wait for 24-36 hours before using. Store bottle in a cool and dark place.

Caution: Do not use Thyme essential oil if you have sensitive skin because it may cause irritation. This is the reason it's at a low concentration. Also, avoid eucalyptus if you have epilepsy or high blood pressure.

Colds

The symptoms of a cold include a sore throat, stuffed-up, runny nose, dry cough and sneezing. Flu is much more serious than a cold, but tends to display similar symptoms.

2 drops lavender

2 drops eucalyptus

2 drops rosemary

2 teaspoons milk or cream

What To Do

1. Add oils to cream or milk.

2. Pour into a warm bath and enjoy.

Colds & Flu Home Spray

1 drop Pine essential oil

1 drop Cinnamon essential oil

1 drop Eucalyptus essential oil

1 drop Cloves essential oil

1 drop Niaouli essential oil

500 ml water

1. Mix the oils in the water and place in a spray can.

2. Shake well to mix the oils well and spray the home.

Anti-Flu Bath

Flu is a severe form of cold. It causes body aches, high fever, chills, exhaustion and muscle sores. Flu viruses are more infectious, more harmful and often stronger than those of colds. They are highly contagious as well.

4 drops Tea tree oil

1 drop of Lemon oil

3 drops Lavender oil

What To Do

Add these oils to a warm bath.

After bath, also massage by combining these oils:

Anti- Flu Massage

3 drops Tea tree oil

2 drops Eucalyptus oil

10 ml Evening primrose oil

Cold Sores Quick Fix

Cold sores are small painful blisters around the lips. They are caused by an outbreak of herpes simplex virus that shows up when stress levels are high. They are called cold sores because the sores usually accompany colds.

1. Use 2 drops Tea tree oil neat or Calendula oil, Chamomile oil or Geranium essential oil diluted in carrier oil.

2. Apply directly onto sore to relieve the pain and swelling.

Cold Sores Blend

4 drops Geranium Essential Oil

2 drops Chamomile Essential Oils

3 drops Tea Tree Essential Oils

1 drop Lavender Essential Oils

10 ml Aloe Vera Gel

What To Do

1. To a 10 ml glass jar, add the Aloe Vera Gel to fill 2/3 of jar.

2. Add the essential oils and mix with spoon. Now fill jar and remix.

3. Apply as prevention when the tingling feeling start or apply direct onto sore to encourage healing.

Kid's Cold Cure

10 drops Lavender

10 drops Eucalyptus

10 drops Tea Tree

<u>What To Do</u>

1. Combine all oils. Put 3 drops of mixture in a diffuser at bedtime.

2. For heavy congestion, put 2 drops of the mixture on cotton piece and tuck it inside the child's pillowcase at night.

3. Put 2 to 5 drops in a bath. The steam will help to clear the nasal passages and help your child to rest.

Nasal Inhaler
For Chest Congestion

5 drops of eucalyptus essential oil

1/4 teaspoon of coarse salt

<u>What To Do</u>

1. Put the salt in a small glass vial. Add the essential oil.

2. Open the vial and inhale deeply as needed all through the day.

Ease Sinus Congestion
2 drops Tea Tree

2 drops Eucalyptus

2 drops Peppermint

<u>What To Do</u>

1. Add oils to steaming pot of water.

2. Cover the pot and head immediately with a towel.

3. Inhale for 3 minutes, keeping eyes closed.

Night-Time Colds & Flu Combater

2 drops Lavender

2 drops Tea Tree

<u>What To Do</u>

1. Add oils to a steaming bowl of water.

2. Let the steam diffuses into the room.

3. Alternatively, add oils to a tea candle diffuser.

SKIN INJURIES & BOO-BOOS

Blisters

Blisters are painful swelling on the skin. It is caused by fluid accumulation underneath the skin. Once the blister bursts, the exposed tissue beneath could become infected. Injury, burning, an insect sting, scalding or chafing could result in blisters.

<u>What To Do</u>

1. Simply apply a drop of tea tree oil or lavender onto the blister.

2. Carefully but thoroughly pat in.

Grazes

Children will always run around and may hurt themselves. Protect them from infection when grazes occur.

<u>What To Do</u>

1. Take out the splinter.

2. Bath all dirt thoroughly by using 10 drops lavender, tea tree, lemon or Eucalyptus in a bowl of warm water.

3. Let the damaged skin remain open in the fresh air. If there is danger of re-infection, make sure you cover-up.

Emergency Burn Wash/Compress

5 drops lavender oil

1 pint water, about 50°F

<u>What To Do</u>

1. Add the oil to the water, stirring well to disperse the oil.

2. Soak a soft cloth in the water and then apply to the burn. Let it stay for 5-10 minutes. Repeat process twice.

3. Alternatively, immerse the burned area directly in the water for 5 minutes.

Bruise

A bruise is a skin discoloration that occurs when blood leaks from damaged blood vessels into the surrounding tissues under the skin. Bruises usually heal naturally but you could use the remedy below for an extra boost.

5 drops Calendula oil

2 drops Fennel oil

1 drop Cypress oil

10 ml Grape seed oil

<u>What To Do</u>

1. Dilute essential oils in carrier oil and massage the affected area.

Minor Burns

2 drops lavender

<u>What To Do</u>

1. Apply ice cold water immediately to the burn for 10 minutes.

2. Apply 2 drops neat lavender onto it.

Insect Bites

1. Remove the sting by applying a few drops of neat lavender oil to it

Insect Repellent Spray

2 ounces distilled water

1.5 ounces witch hazel or vodka

25 drops peppermint oil

30 drops citronella oil

15 drops tea tree oil

1 teaspoon of jojoba oil (optional but if you add this, add only 1 oz of witch hazel or vodka)

<u>What To Do</u>

1. Add the vodka or witch hazel to a 4 oz clean spray bottle filled with distilled or boiled water.

2. Add the essential oils and shake thoroughly. Spray onto clothing and/or exposed skin but avoid the eyes and mucous membranes.

3. Reapply as needed. Store it in a dark bottle and away from sunlight or heat. This makes 4 ounces

Antiseptic Cream
For cuts and wounds

20 drops Lavender Essential Oil

15 drops Tea Tree Essential Oil

15 drops Geranium Essential Oil

43 ml Base Cream

What To Do

1. Add the Base Cream to a fill 2/3 of 50 ml dark colored glass jar.

2. Add essential oils, mixing with a spoon. Fill jar

3. Use directly onto injury, cover with bandage for quicker healing.

Wounds

Wounds must be sterilized to prevent infection.

2 drops Tea Tree oil

5 drops Lavender oil

500 ml warm water

<u>What To Do</u>

1. Combine oils in water and bathe the wound area.

2. Cover up the wound by dropping 3 drops of Lavender oil on a piece of gauze and then placing it over the cut.

3. Renew two times daily. On the third day, expose the wound to air if possible.

Bleeding

Bleeding should always be taken seriously, regardless of what kind it is. An adult usually has about 5 liter of blood. Even the loss of 1 liter can be fatal.

For a small open wound:

1 drop Chamomile oil

1 drop Geranium oil

1 drop Lemon oil

1 drop Tea Tree oil

1. Combine and apply as a compress.

Cuts Spray
To reduce the risk of infection

6 drops eucalyptus oil

12 drops tea tree oil

6 drops of lemon oil

2 oz distilled water

What To Do

1. Combine all the ingredients, shaking well before each use.

2. Dispense as needed from a spray bottle. Use on minor cuts, burns or abrasions to speed healing and prevent infection.

Boils

Boils are abscesses usually found at the buttocks or underarms. Fever and fatigue can be associated with boils as well.

<u>Ingredients</u>

2 drops Tea tree oil

2 drops Lavender oil

1 drop Juniper oil

200 ml hot water

<u>What To Do</u>

1. Dilute the essential oils in the hot water.

2. For severe inflammation, add 1 drop Chamomile oil.

3. Bathe the area two times daily.

4. Alternatively, apply undiluted tea tree or lavender oil to the area using a cotton bud.

Anti- Abscess Compress

An abscess is typically caused by bacteria and forms around a hair follicle. Generally, however, it is a pus- filled cavity where the skin becomes red and swollen and later develops into a throbbing elevated lump.

2 drops Tea Tree essential oil

2 drops Lavender essential oil

2 drops Chamomile essential oil

Combine and apply to the area of swelling twice daily.

HEADACHES

A headache is simply a pain in the head but the severity of the discomfort varies to a great extent. Headaches are symptomatic. The underlying cause could be stress, tension, fatigue, allergies or blocked sinuses. Others include drug overuse, adverse reaction to medication and seasonal changes.

Fast Fix Remedy

3 drops lavender essential oils

2 drops peppermint essential oils

<u>What To Do</u>

1. Add oils to fold-up tissue.

2. Inhale slowly and deeply in 3 long breaths.

3. Repeat three times.

Anti- Headache Blend

1 drop Peppermint oil

3 drops Lavender oil

3 drops Jojoba oil

1 drop Bergamot oil

What To Do

1. Mix oils and massage around the temples or into the base of the skull.

Tension/ Nervous Headache Mix

1 drop Clary sage oil

3 drops of Lavender oil

2 drops of Jojoba oil

1 drop Chamomile oil

What To Do

1. Mix oils and massage around the temples or into the base of the skull.

Headache Balm

1 tablespoon Beeswax, grated

1/4 cup Shea Butter

1/4 teaspoon (or 1 capsule) Vitamin E

1 tablespoon Grapeseed oil

8 drops Lavender essential oil

1 drop Chamomile essential oil

1 drop Jasmine essential oil

<u>What To Do</u>

1. Place the beeswax, Shea butter & grapeseed oil in a double boiler over a low heat until melted.

2. Remove from heat; add the essential oils and the vitamin E. Pour into a dark glass jar and store in a cool, dark place.

3. Rub onto back of your neck and your temples to ease pain and soothe tension.

STOMACH RELIEF

Diarrhea

Diarrhea is the frequent and excessive discharge of the bowel movement, signaling that something is not right with the system. It could be caused by eating spicy foods, undigested vegetables, unripe fruits, excessive food consumption, eating too fast and drinking unclean water.

A massage oil to help ease diarrhea

2 drops Lavender essential oil

2 drops Peppermint essential oil

2 drops Eucalyptus essential oil

2 drops Chamomile essential oil

2 drops Geranium essential oil

10 ml vegetable carrier oil

Combine and rub over the abdomen area.

Hiccups

Hiccups are not meant to last for a long time otherwise they can be very painful.

<u>What To Do</u>

1. Place 1 drop Chamomile essential oil in a brown paper bag.

2. Hold the bag over your nose and mouth.

3. Breathe in slowly and deeply through your nose.

Stomach Massage

For indigestion

2 drops Cinnamon

4 drops Peppermint

6 drops Mandarin

2 tablespoons carrier oil

<u>What To Do</u>

1. Dilute essential oils with the carrier oil.

2. Massage onto stomach.

Nausea Instant Remedy

The underlying cause of nausea can be physiological, psychological or both. Reasons such as disgusting smells, hangovers, bad digestion, food poisoning, motion sickness, early pregnancy and tonsillitis could contribute to nausea.

1 drop of Lavender essential oil

1 drop Peppermint essential oil

1 drop Basil essential oil

2 teaspoons (10ml) carrier oil of choice

<u>What To Do</u>

1. Combine all the oils. Massage over your abdomen very gently.

2. Cup your hands over your mouth & nose and then inhale a few times slowly. Wash your hands.

Motion Sickness

1. Add 2 drops lavender or bergamot essential oil to a handkerchief and sniff.

2. Get enough fresh air.

Heartburn

Heartburn is an uncomfortable burning pain in the lower chest. It often occurs after a meal when the stomach acids flows back into the esophagus' lower end.

2 drops Eucalyptus oil

 2 drops Fennel oil

1 drop Peppermint oil

1 teaspoon (5ml) Grape seed oil

<u>What To Do</u>

1. Dilute the essential oils in the carrier oil

2. Rub the upper abdominal area with this mixture.

Bladder Infection Oil

6 drops tea tree oil

8 drops juniper berry or cypress oil

2 drops fennel oil

6 drops bergamot oil

2 ounces vegetable oil

<u>What To Do</u>

1. Combine all ingredients. Massage once a day over the bladder area.

2. For prevention, add 1 tablespoon of this mixture to your bath.

Bladder Infection Sitz Bath

5 drops lavender oil

5 drops rosemary oil

<u>What To Do</u>

1. Add the essential oils to hot bath

2. Sit for 5-10 minutes in a tub with the hot water up to the waist.

3. Next, switch to a tub of cold water for at 1-2 minute. Do 2-5 rounds.

4. Do this treatment daily or at least two times a week.

PAINS

For Rheumatism & Arthritis

3 drops Chamomile

3 drops Lavender

3 drops Yarrow

3 drops Eucalyptus

8 ounces sweet-almond oil

Add the essential oils to almond oil

Massage into affected areas.

Massage Oil For Abdominal Pain

Abdominal pain may be caused by eating too fast, digestive problems or menstruation.

1 drop of Chamomile oil

1 drop Peppermint oil

1 drop Clove oil

5 ml Carrier oil of choice

What To Do

1. Dilute the essential oils in the carrier.

2. Massage the stomach area gently in a clockwise motion.

3. If the pain persists, seek medical advice.

Massage Oil Remedy

2 drops Thyme oil

3 drops Eucalyptus oil

1 drop Pine oil

1 teaspoon Jojoba oil

<u>What To Do</u>

1. Dilute essential oils in Jojoba

2. Massage the back and chest.

Cramp

Cramp is the sudden painful involuntary contraction of a muscle or group of muscles.

3 drops Geranium essential oil

5 ml Evening primrose oil

<u>What To Do</u>

1. Combine oils and massage on the legs.

Bedsores

Bedsores also called pressure sores occur when the body is subjected to constant pressure and irritation. The sores become painful ulcerations and are usually found on the buttocks, elbows and heels of people, especially, bedridden patients.

Bedsore Massage Oil

3 drops Chamomile or Geranium oil

2 drops Tea tree oil

2 drops Lavender oil

4 drops Wheat germ oil

2 drops Frankincense oil

20 ml Evening primrose oil

What To Do

1. Mix all ingredients together.

2. Gently massage the affected area.

3. May be used before bedsore develops.

ORAL HEALTH

Mouth Ulcers

Mouth ulcers are tiny open sores in the mouth, tongue, the roof of the mouth or the mucus membrane inside the cheeks and lips. Ulcers can last from 2 days-3weeks but they heal spontaneously and leave no scar.

<u>What To Do</u>

1. Put 2 drops Tea Tree oil in cotton bud & apply neat dipped to the ulcer.

2. Alternatively, make a mouthwash by adding 2 drops of Tea Tree oil and 5ml salt to 500 ml warm and boiled water.

3. Power Mouthwash

   2 drops Thyme oil

   2 drops Geranium oil

   2 drops Peppermint oil

   2 drops Lemon oil

   2 drops Tea tree oil

   1 glass warm water

   10 ml brandy

Combine ingredients& Use as mouthwash. Swish around the mouth and spit.

Gum Strengthener

Firm up gums and prevent gum disease.

1 drop Cinnamon

1 teaspoon of vodka

2 tablespoons of water

<u>What To Do</u>

1. Add the essential oil to vodka and water. Shake the mixture thoroughly.

2. Swish your toothbrush in this mixture. Brush your teeth as usual.

Bad Breath

Bad breath is embarrassing. It could be a symptom of a root problem such as indigestion or improper toxic elimination by the liver or kidney. It could be caused by plaque buildup, decomposing food between the teeth, cigarette smoking and ingestion of strong foods such as garlic and onions.

4 drops Lavender oil

125 ml warm water

5 ml Brandy

<u>What To Do</u>

1. Dilute the oil in the brandy and water and use as mouthwash.

2. Swirl around the mouth after brushing and flossing. Rinse and spit out.

3. Use as needed.

Chapped Lips

Chapped lips can be very painful. It is difficult to keep from licking your sore lips but this process usually increases the pain.

1 drop Chamomile oil

1 drop Neroli oil

2 drops Rose oil

2 drops Geranium oil

20 ml Aloe Vera oil

Mix all the ingredients together in a roller bottle. Apply to lips to ease pain and foster healing.

Toothache

Toothache is usually very painful. It can be regarded as one of the worst pains caused by a minor ailment.

What To Do

1. Put 1 drop of clove essential oil on a cotton bud.

2. Place the cotton bud on the gum around the tooth.

2. Alternatively, place into the crevices on either side.

Massage Oil For Toothache

1 drop Lemon oil

1 drop Clove oil

3 drops Chamomile oil

5 ml vegetable oil

What To Do

1. Dilute in vegetable oil.

2. Massage the cheek and jawbone.

SKIN CARE REMEDIES

For Stretch Marks

3 drops Yarrow

1 teaspoon carrier of choice

Mix and daily rub on the affected areas.

Sunburn Soother

20 drops of lavender oil

1 tablespoon vinegar

200 IU vitamin E oil

4 ounces aloe Vera juice

What To Do

1. Combine all the ingredients. Shake thoroughly before using.

2. store in a spritzer bottle and use as needed.

3. Keep the spray in the refrigerator for extra coolness relief coolness will

Gentle Wart Removal

Eliminate warts and prevent future outbreaks

1 drop Lemon essential oil (per wart)

Apply undiluted to the affected area directly. Do this several times a day for at 4-5 weeks.

Blemish Blocker

Dab a little of this highly effective mix on your pimple; do not use too often because it may dry out your skin

10 drops Lemon

10 drops Lavender

10 drops Tea Tree

<u>What To Do</u>

1. Combine oils in a dark glass container.

2. Use a cotton swab to apply tiny amounts to skin blemishes.

3. Note: although lemon is not usually applied neat, unlike lavender and tea tree, it is safe for spot-treating" purpose in this preparation.

Easy Facial Toner

5 drops Lavender

5 drops Yarrow

4 oz. Springwater

<u>What To Do</u>

1. Combine all the ingredients. Use as a facial toner.

2. Alternately, add only the essential oils to a simple moisturizer or lotion.

Facial Toner

For oily skin

6 drops juniper berry oil

12 drops lemongrass oil

2 drops ylang ylang oil

1 ounce witch hazel lotion

1 ounce aloe Vera gel

<u>What To Do</u>

1. Combine all the ingredients. Use as a facial toner.

Intensive Blemish Treatment

12 drops tea tree oil

1/2 teaspoon of powdered Oregon grape root, powdered

800 units vitamin E (optional)

A few drops of water

<u>What To Do</u>

1. Add together the herb powder and essential oil, stirring to make a paste.

2. Apply directly as a mask on the blemished area.

3. Allow the paste to dry and remain on your skin for 20-30 minutes, then rinse off.

4. Repeat again before bedtime, if you wish.

FEVER

A fever is an unusually high body temperature that is often caused by a viral or bacterial infection. Symptoms include shivering, apathy, headache, upward turning of the eyes and dullness. If fevers get too high they could lead to cause seizures or even delirium and this can affect the brain.

Fever Massage Blend

1 drop Rosemary essential oil

2 drops Eucalyptus essential oil

1 drop Tea Tree essential oil

2 drops Peppermint essential oil

2 drops Lavender essential oil

1 drop Black pepper essential oil

15 ml Evening primrose oil

What To Do

1. Add oils together.

2. Massage the top of hands, back of neck, temples and soles of feet.

EYE CARE

Sty

Sty is a temporal swelling on the eyelid. It can develop on the outside as a red sore or itchy spot, which swells and then forms a yellow or pink head. An internal sty is even more painful. The yellowish head is only noticeable when the eyelid is lifted.

1 drop Chamomile essential oil

10 ml rosewater

<u>What To Do</u>

1. Add together and boil.

2. Once cooled, place in a container and shake thoroughly.

3. Strain through a coffee filter and then use the strained mixture to make the compress.

Conjunctivitis Compress

Conjunctivitis is an infection of the conjunctiva. It can be caused by viruses, bacteria, sand, dust or smoke. Symptoms include redness, itching, irritation, burning and tearing.

1 drop of Chamomile oil

5 ml Witch hazel

30 ml Rosewater

<u>What To Do</u>

Combine ingredients and leave for 7-9 hours. Strain
through a paper coffee filter. Use as a compress on the
closed eyelids.

EAR, NOSE & THROAT

Catarrh

Catarrh is the overproduction and secretion of mucus from the throat and nose. The causes of include colds, flu, bronchitis, hay fever, sinusitis and rhinitis.

1 drop Thyme oil

1 drop Eucalyptus oil

<u>What To Do</u>

1. Drop oils in a bowl of hot water.

2. Drape a towel over your head

3. Inhale for 10 minutes.

Hay Fever

Hay fever is an allergic reaction to pollen or dust. They occur quite spontaneously and usually affect the eyes and the upper respiratory tract. The symptoms include itching eyes, watering eyes, sneezing and runny nose.

<u>What To Do</u>

1. Put 2-3 drops of Tea Tree, Niaouli or Eucalyptus oil on a handkerchief and inhale when an attack occurs.

2. Make a room spray using diluted Eucalyptus oil

Catarrh Rub

3 drops of Tea tree oil

3 drops Rosemary oil

3 drops of Eucalyptus oil

15 ml Evening primrose oil

<u>What To Do</u>

Combine and rub on the chest and the back area.

Pain Relief For Earache

Ear pain is often caused by an infection in the middle-ear. Some of the symptoms are: shooting pains in the ear(s), noises in the ear, fever, a feeling of fullness in the ear, vomiting, nausea and diarrhea.

1 drop Clove oil

5 ml Grape seed oil

<u>What To Do</u>

1. Mix and massage around the ear and neck.

2. If the ear infection was caused by a throat infection, just add 2 drops of Tea tree to a glass of boiled water and then gargle every 2 hours.

Sinusitis Steam Inhalation

Sinusitis is an inflammation of the sinus lining. It could be caused by a flu, cold, tonsillitis, poor mouth hygiene or allergies. The symptoms include nosebleed, nasal congestion, ear pain, fatigue, headache, a mild fever, pain around the eyes or cough.

1 drop Eucalyptus oil

2 drops Peppermint oil

2 drops Rosemary oil

1 drop Thyme oil

Use steam inhalation with these oils.

Massage Oil For Sinusitis

2 drops Eucalyptus oil

3 drops Rosemary oil

2 drops Peppermint oil

1 drop Tea tree oil

3 drops Geranium oil

10 ml carrier oil

What To Do

1. Add essential oils to carrier oil of choice.

2. Massage the nose, around the nose, neck, forehead, cheekbones and in front and behind the ears.

Nosebleed

For a nosebleed without injury or a broken nose, use the remedy below. However, if there is injury or broken nose, see a doctor.

1 drop Lavender oil

3 drops Lemon oil

<u>What To Do</u>

1. Combine oils in a tissue and inhale.

2. Apply an icepack as well.

BODY ACHES & PAINS

Muscle Pain

2 drops Rosemary

2 drops Lavender

4 teaspoons carrier oil of choice

<u>What To Do</u>

1. Combine oils and massage gently onto affected area.

Nerve Pain Oil

Nerves register pain, so when they are damaged, the condition is usually painful. Although injured nerves regenerate slowly, aromatherapy treatments can help to speed up the process.

3 drops marjoram oil

4 drops chamomile oil

2 drops lavender oil

3 drops helichrysum oil (optional)

1 oz vegetable oil

<u>What To Do</u>

1. Combine all ingredients. Apply daily as needed for pain relief.

Back Pain Massage

Back problems can make daily life a misery. Severe pain could be caused by problems with the bone, tendons, ligaments or even a pulled muscle. Other factors that affect the back muscles include, lack of exercise, obesity and incorrect posture. Relieve back pain naturally with this aromatherapy massage:

4 drops cardamom oil

4 drops ginger oil

4 drops wintergreen oil

1 tablespoon sweet oil

<u>What To Do</u>

1. Blend oils and soothingly massage.

Aromatherapy Bath

Soothe tired, aching muscles

8-10 drops essential oils added directly to warm bath water. Soak for 15-20 minutes.

LOWER BLOOD PRESSURE

1 drop Ylang-ylang

2 drops of Clary-Sage

Place these 3 drops on a tissue and inhale.

EMOTIONAL HEALTH

Insomnia Blend

Insomnia means sleeplessness. It is usually caused by anxiety or stress or by physical problems like menopause or pre-menstrual tension. Sleep deprivation may eventually lead to depression chronic agitation, headaches and dizziness. Aromatherapy usually helps.

10 drops lavender oil

15 drops bergamot oil

2 drops ylang ylang oil

10 drops sandalwood oil

3 drops frankincense (optional)

4 ounces vegetable oil

<u>What To Do</u>

1. Combine all ingredients and use combination as massage oil.

2. Put 2 teaspoons in your bath.

3. Alternatively use in a diffuser without the vegetable oil.

Insomnia Remedy

1. Half an hour before bedtime, take a warm bath to which has been added 2-3drops of Lavender or Neroli oil.

2. Alternatively, massage the body with 2-3 drops of Lavender, Clary sage, Ylang ylang or Sandalwood essential oil diluted in carrier oil.

Jetlag

Jetlag occurs when your body's psychological and physiological rhythms are disrupted due to long flights taken. The symptoms include sleep disturbance, fatigue, aching or swollen feet and nausea.

What To Do

1. During the flight, massage your feet with 1 drop of Geranium, Grapefruit or Basil oil diluted with a dash of carrier oil.

2. On arrival, put 10 drops of Lavender oil in your hand and rub on the torso to stay alert and then shower immediately.

3. Revive your mind and body by adding the oils below to a warm bath. Enjoy

2 drops Peppermint essential oil

1 drop Bergamot essential oil

1 drop Rosemary essential oil

1 drop Geranium essential oil

2 drops Neroli essential oil

Release Sexual Energy
2 drop of Sandalwood

2 drops Rosemary

2 drops Jasmine

2 teaspoons jojoba oil

Combine the essential oils in a simmer pot or diffuser.

Comfort the Bereaved
Console the grief-stricken

5 drops Sandalwood

3 drops Rose-Otto

2 teaspoons of jojoba oil

Combine and use as massage

Fatigue Fader
Feel refreshed & renewed

2 drops Lemon

2 drops Peppermint

1. In a small bowl, combine essential oils.

2. Dip a cold, moist cloth into the mixture. Lie down; drape cloth across your forehead and temples.

3. Breathe in through your nose and breathe out through your mouth. Do so for 15- 30 minutes.

Concentration Spray
Fight after-lunch sleepiness with this remedy

2 drops Peppermint

3 drops Lemon

3 drops Rosemary

2 cups water

What To Do

1. Add the oils to water and spray around your office or home.